Fit 4 Life

Overcoming the obstacles to our wellbeing

At Work Edition

MARK COWLING

ISBN-10: 1729656072
ISBN-13:978-1729656075

DEDICATION

Thanks to Tony Vino for friendship and wisdom.

CONTENTS

	Introduction	Pg 7
1	Recognising the parts –Mind, Heart, Will	Pg 8
2	Success as wellbeing vs standard of living	Pg 9
3	Success requires values –Courage as the first	Pg 10
4	Being strong for life –Overcoming habits and holds	Pg 11
5	Dealing with Anger	Pg 12
6	Forgiveness	Pg 13
7	Dealing with Desires-Discipline of self control	Pg 14
8	Balance for life –Work, Living, Playing, Giving	Pg 15
9	Managing Money	Pg 17
10	Goals	Pg 19
11	Healthy Relationships Part 1–Why is staying together so hard?	Pg 21
12	Healthy Relationships Part 2–Why is work such a nightmare?	Pg 22

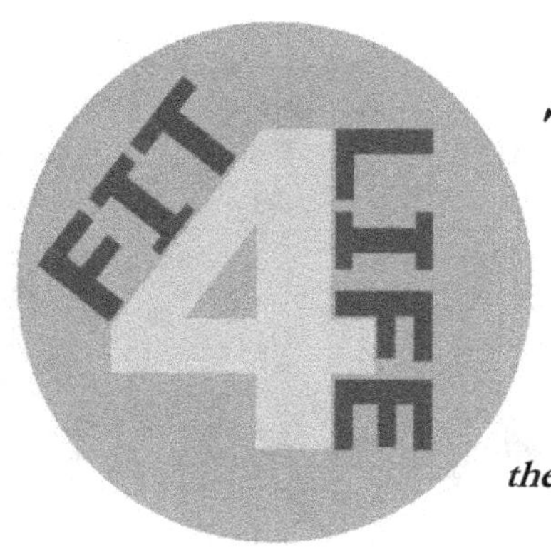

The Fit4Life Course

**Overcoming obstacles
to our health and wellbeing.**

*"In the workplace people are our greatest
asset but often relationships aren't working and
there is a lack of wellbeing."*

*"Health is a state of
complete physical, mental
and social well-being and
not merely the absence of
disease or infirmity. "*

World Health Organisation

Are you fit and healthy? Do you know what being healthy looks like?...
Experience tells us that there are a great many opposing forces in our world that challenge our health and wellbeing both in the workplace and in family life. Wellbeing of people is a vital moral purpose as well as being integral to long term performance in the workplace. When we spend such a big part of our lives at work, wellbeing deserves to be made a priority, by us and by the organisations we belong to and work for. Yet, for many organisations, embracing this ideal requires a social and cultural transformation, a movement away from a culture of institution towards being more like a family -a group that values emotional intelligence and community for the sake of wellbeing. This is wholeness and it's life giving rather than life draining.

Managing people and being part of work groups comes with thrills and spills. It's a thrill when things go well — "well-managed workgroups are more profitable (44% higher), more productive (50% higher), and have higher degrees of customer loyalty (50% higher)". The spills are all too familiar leading to the opposite outcomes. Research shows that poor relationships with the boss is the overwhelming challenge in the workplace -50% of people who leave their job do so because they are so unhappy with their boss. Whilst managers are often taught about the functional elements (see The Gallup 12 Elements in Session 12) of managing which support performance, they often neglect a healthy relationship, which includes appreciating how people are different and having understanding and concern for the wellbeing of others. Neglecting this human-side is like running using just one leg.

This course covers 12 foundations for wellbeing, helping people put wellbeing into practice, developing them as role models with a shared vocabulary and personal stories, making them people fit to follow and fit to lead.

For leaders; the material can work well with medium sized groups, but is ideal for a group of 4 plus the leader as it can aid more open sharing and discussion. We recommend pens and paper to allow people to take notes and doodle. More information including Youtube links are available at www.fit4lifecourse.blogspot.com

Inside
- 1. Recognising the parts –Mind, Heart, Will
- 2. Success as wellbeing vs standard of living
- 3. Success requires values –Courage as the first
- 4. Being strong for life –Overcoming habits and holds
- 5. Dealing with Anger
- 6. Forgiveness
- 7. Dealing with Desires-Discipline of self control

Outside
- 8. Balance for life –Work, Living, Playing, Giving
- 9. Managing Money
- 10. Goals

Outwards
- 11. Healthy Relationships Part 1–Why is staying together so hard?
- 12. Healthy Relationships Part 2–Why is work such a nightmare?

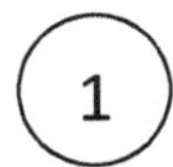

(1) Recognising the parts –Mind, Heart, Will
An introduction to Wellbeing

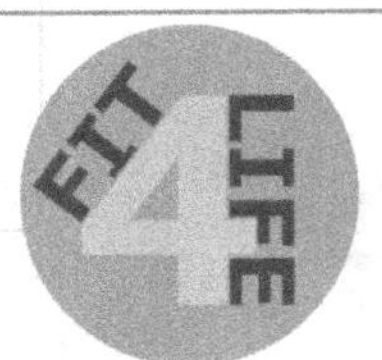

Aim: To understand wellbeing definition: "state of health physically, mentally, socially". Wellbeing definition (below) recognises that there are three parts to us: Mind =knowledge. Heart =seat of emotions. Soul = Will

Icebreaker: Take it in turns to tell the group three things about you – two must be true and one false. The group has to decide which is which.

Exercise:
i) Write your name & what it means – google it on i-phone if you don't know
ii) Draw a graph (1-10 on vertical and your age from 0-now on horizontal). Plot a line of how you have felt about yourself and your life through time. Note the Banksy tweet picture below.
iii) Write down some ambitions "'One thing I want to do before I die…'.

These three exercises illustrate the parts to us: Mind =knowledge. Heart =seat of emotions. Soul = Will

Discussion: Wellbeing is more about health of mind heart and will (as defined below) rather than standard of living. The quotes below describe some opposition to wellbeing. What does this look like in your experience?

In the workplace: "The Invisible Hand has dropped the common good" is a quote from Jim Wallis using Adam Smith's metaphor for Capitalism that says we have lost the concern for people's wellbeing in our economy.

In the family: "40% of cohabiting relationships break up before the first child is five years old," is a quote from Nicky Gumbel that illustrates how unstable family life has become. What's more, absent fathers hugely increase the chances of children dropping out of school, having a drug addiction, committing suicide and facing prison sentences.

"Health is a state of complete physical, mental and social well-being and not merely the absence of disease or infirmity. "

World Health Organisation

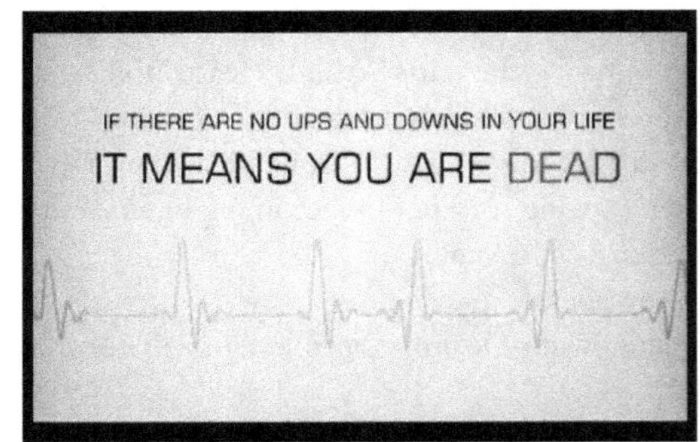

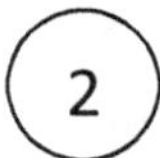 **Wellbeing brings success in life**
Wellbeing vs standard of living

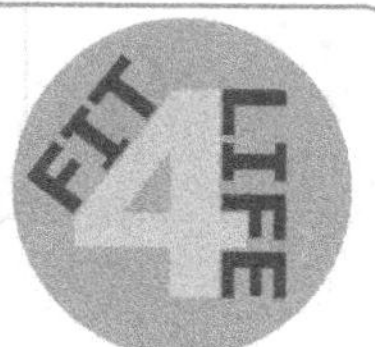

Aim: To appreciate that wellbeing can bring quality of life.

Recap: Last week's session.

Icebreaker 1: Ask people to score how they feel out of ten (remembering Banksy's picture in session one). Then ask them to give one word (if possible) to explain why they scored their feelings with that number. This is a recommended icebreaker for every session.

Icebreaker 2: Put a bag of coloured sweets (M&Ms) in a container and allocate one of the questions to each of the colours. Get the group to take turns to take a coloured sweet randomly from a container and then depending what colour sweet they draw out, answer one the following categories;
i) what's your favourite movie? ii) tell the group a surprising fact about yourself? iii) what's your favourite cheese? iv) what's your favourite place? v) if you had a time travel machine, who would you most like to meet?

Exercises:
1) Write down some answers to these questions:
i) What is success?
ii) One thing I wish my friends/family understood about me is…
iii) One thing I dream about for my kids is…'

2) Have a look through the newspapers and find good and bad examples of success.

Discussion:
Discuss one or all of these quotes;
"Happiness = someone to love, a job to do and something to look forward to."

"Emotional intelligence (mastering your emotions) is a predictor of success more than IQ"

Proverbs 16:13: "Kings [Leaders] take pleasure in honest lips; they value the one who speaks what is right" illustrates that "Wisdom (the good application of knowledge+emotions+will) = success

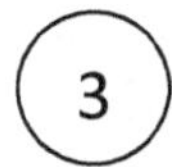

(3) How to develop wellbeing
the role of virtue

Aim: To appreciate that wellbeing needs to be constructed by building virtues in our lives

Recap: Last week's session

Icebreaker Picture Whispers -like Chinese Whispers but by drawing pictures instead of using voices. A word is written on page one of a notepad, then the first participant draws the word on page two before handing it on to the next person to draw on page three, referencing only the previous page i.e. not page one! On completion the notebook is read backwards with each participant attempting to explain what they were drawing. To keep everybody engaged, you can run multiple notepads, with different words, all at once.

Exercises:
The British army is a high performing team committed to peace making; it's a team that deals with the very worst of life (wars), but demands the very best performance of people. The army knows that wellbeing is crucial for the success of its employees and has 6 core values.

Write the 6 values below onto separate pieces of paper and randomly arrange them on the table. *Courage, Discipline, Respect, Integrity, Loyalty, Selfless commitment.*

Ask the group which value from the "CDRILS" list of British army values & standards is rated as #1 by the Army inc. Winston Churchill. Discuss the answer that Courage is rated #1 because "everything else flows from courage". Why? Because there will always be opposition to good in our world and courage is needed to overcome the opposition.

Discussion:
Discuss one or all of these quotes;

i) *"Physical Courage without moral courage can be a dangerous thing because it can lead us into "stupid bravery"."*

ii) *"For some of us, trying to rescue someone from a burning building is easier than facing our emotions involved in difficult relationships – why?"*

iii) *"Moral Courage is like a muscle. It needs exercising to grow strong – how do we do that?"*
One example is when our football team is losing badly we need to keep our heads up and pull together.

Read: Psalm 1:1-6 "..That person is like a tree planted by streams of water, which yields its fruit in season and whose leaf does not wither – whatever they do prospers."

(4) Overcoming holds in our life
getting free from habits and addictions

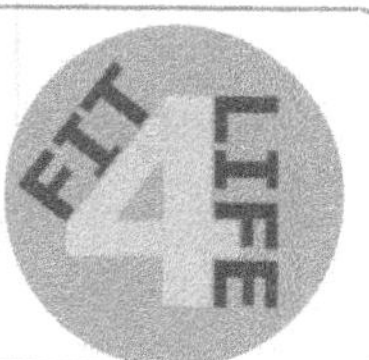

Aim: To appreciate we have desires, habits and behaviours that can be obstacles to our progress and freedom.

Recap: Last week's session

Exercise: Holding an orange, explain that to catch a monkey, some African tribes put an orange inside a coconut and tie the coconut to a tree. There is a small hole in the coconut and when the monkey puts his hand inside to grab the orange, it cannot then pull its hand with the orange in it out. But because it doesn't want to let go of the orange, it is trapped.

Explain that we all have things in our lives that are like that orange and life involves learning to let go of these things. Ask the group to write down the "orange" they are holding on to.

Discuss what the steps to letting go might be. See if the group can guess these 4 recommended steps:

1) Admitting – denial is the biggest obstacle to overcoming our unhelpful habits

2) Desiring to let go –agreeing that life without the "orange" in our life would be preferable

3) Planning boundaries –considering what boundaries need to be put in place to enable us to stay free

4) Setting gatekeepers –determining who we can be accountable to and supported by as we try to live with the boundaries

Overcoming ceremony: Each take it in turns to hold the orange and, if willing, declare what their "orange" issue is and what their next step will be. Others reply "I hear you brother". Burning the pieces of paper with these "orange issues" might also be symbolically helpful.

Read: Romans 7:21-25 which identifies with habits and holds in our lives; *"..So I find this law at work: although I want to do good, evil is right there with me. 22 For in my inner being I delight in God's law; 23 but I see another law at work in me, waging war against the law of my mind and making me a prisoner of the law of sin at work within me. 24 What a wretched man I am! Who will rescue me from this body that is subject to death?" [You can read on for Paul's answer]*

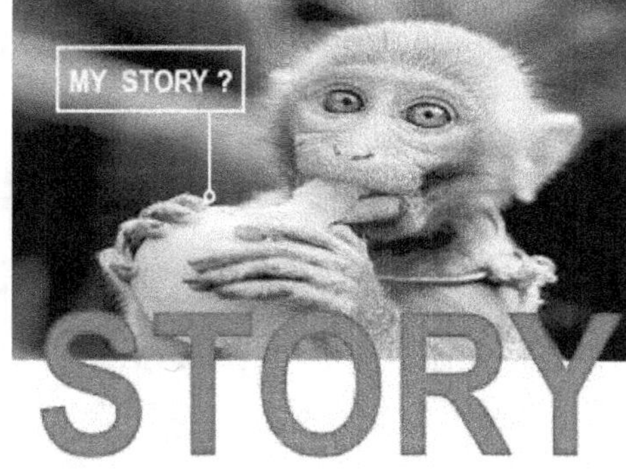

5 Dealing with anger

...in a healthy way

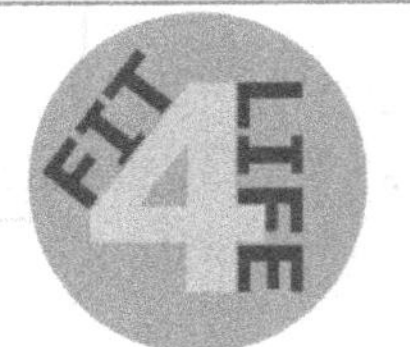

Aim: To learn about anger and how to respond to it in a healthy way.

Recap: Last week's session

Icebreaker: Looking at Premier League football what things do players, managers and spectators get angry about regularly?

Anger Fact File:

i) Adrenalin is released when we experience anger which leads to a "fight or flight" response

ii) Our culture affects the way we behave emotionally eg Gazza crying in World Cup is OK but us crying at work is more awkward. We might cry at a funeral, but less likely to cry in prison. It is probably more socially acceptable to cry when you are drunk in a pub than reading a paper on a bus. Perhaps women deal with others crying better- do they have the skill of empathy?

iii) There are times when we are weaker at dealing with our emotions (including anger). Those occasions spell an acronym H.A.L.T. –Hungry, Angry, Lonely, Tired.

iv) Dramatic exploding anger is sometimes a cry for help. If we are not heard anger can implode and lead to depression.

v) When we don't deal with our anger in a healthy way, we can try to repair relationships by saying sorry. It's not a weakness for children to see us say sorry to them.

Exercises:

1) What do people do when they're angry? *Is lack of control part of it?*

2) Is anger good or bad? *Anger is natural. Channelling anger is key.*

3) In studies domestic abuse is said to increase more than 30% on match days match days – why? *We displace/transfer anger into convenient/alternative situations. N.B. Some people express anger at home but rarely at work, some people do the opposite.*

4) Write down some things that make you angry. Then write the feelings you had. Can you assess/diagnose what the root cause is?

5) Read the anger fact file (above) and discuss.

6) Ask the group for helpful ideas for when you're about to explode...*some listed below*

Count to ten – or 100 if you're really mad

Go into a different room until you've cooled off (especially if you're with babies/children)

Imagine a relaxing scene or listen to some chilled music.

Repeat what the other person has said and ask for some time to consider it.

Breathe in slowly for five seconds and out for five seconds. Keep going until you feel calmer.

Pray! Ask God to help you keep in control and feel more peaceful. Ask him to show you the wise way to deal with the situation.

Speak to a mature and trusted friend about your anger and ask for their advice.

Try to reconcile quickly. Why might the Bible in *Ephesians 4:26* say *".. 'In your anger do not sin': do not let the sun go down while you are still angry,"*

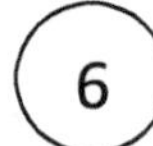

(6) Forgiveness
the power of saying sorry and letting go

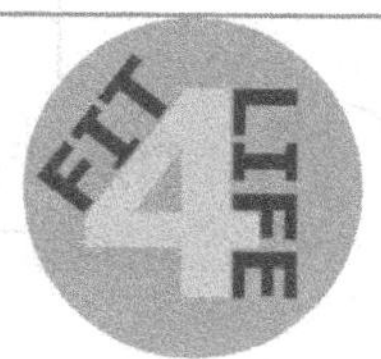

Aim: To learn about the power of forgiveness

Recap: Last week's session

Icebreaker: Ask people to score how they feel out of ten (remembering Banksy's picture in session one). Then ask them to give one word (if possible) to explain why they scored their feelings with that number. This is a recommended icebreaker for every session.

Discussion:

1) Encourage people to say what comes into their heads when they think of the word 'forgiveness'.

2) What does it mean to 'forgive' someone?
The dictionary definition is: 'The act of excusing a mistake or offence'. It highlights that forgiving someone is a deliberate choice/action.

3) Is forgiving someone something you find easy to do?
Very few people find it easy to forgive 100 per cent of the time.
Gandhi once said, "The weak can never forgive. Forgiveness is the attribute of the strong." It takes guts and determination to excuse someone who has hurt or offended us.

Nelson Mandela in the film Invictus speaks to his black security guards about the need to work with the white security guards (who had previously beaten them up under apartheid). Reconciliation in Mandela's Rainbow Nation started with forgiveness in the President's office. Mandela asks "please try Jason"

Corrie Ten Boom after suffering in a Nazi concentration camp felt compelled to forgive the Nazi soldier who asked her forgiveness, describing it as a "mechanical act which was followed by her heart emotion afterwards". Corrie reached beyond herself in this act.

4) Forgiveness is related to loss *(because something has usually been taken from us)*. Loss has a cycle of emotions: i)denial,ii) anger,iii) bargaining,iv) depression, v) acceptance *(forgiveness is part of a healthy "acceptance" state moving forward but we will probably experience the other stages too)*

5) Forgiveness and justice: is making a mends important?

Forgiveness and peace: Knowing we are forgiven is life giving. Especially in our own family. Is our desire for being a peacemaker (requiring courage) greater than other desires?
Read: Matthew 18:21-35: What was the difference between what the king in Jesus' story did, and what the first official did? - Why did the king get so cross with the official whose debt he cancelled? - At the end of the story, Jesus explains that the king who forgave the official is a picture of God. What does this mean for us and how we treat people who have wronged us? Does God, as forgiver, help you?

7 **The discipline of self control**
managing our desires

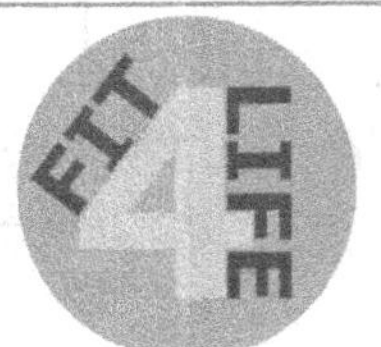

Aim: To learn about the nature of our desires and impulses and how to control them

Recap: Last week's session

Icebreaker: Everybody take a piece of bubble gum and have a competition to seewho can blow the biggest bubble. Measure or visually judge the biggest and applaud the winner.
OR
Guess the size in cm of the world record for the biggest bubble gum bubble. It's 56 cm. Search it on Youtube.

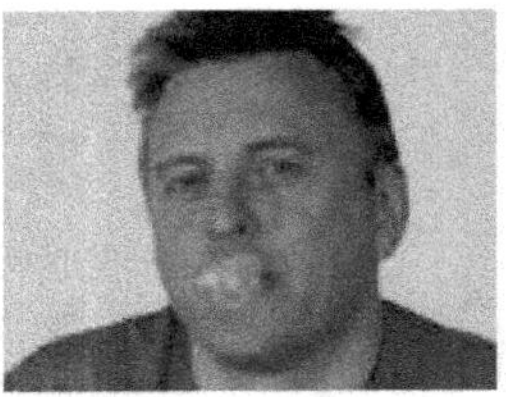

Discussion: The "bubble of desire" grows inside of us sometimes, squashing everything else out of proportion. Especially seen in young children. Violet Beauregard in Charlie and the Chocolate factory was a metaphor of this "bubble of desire" which made her literally inflate!
Reading: Genesis 3:1-7 depicts the ancient human problem of "self control". Genesis 3:6 "..When the woman saw it was pleasing to the eye and also desirable she took some and ate it"

Other than food, what kind of appetites do we experience that develop as desires *(Money, attention, women-lust/comfort/companionship, fame, power, authority, control, relaxation/escape, bonding to overcome loneliness, food, perfection, self-expression)*

What top tips do you have for managing your desires?
o Active thankfulness (reflecting on those less fortunate, "fasting"/going without for a period
o Focus on the goal & stepping stones (ability to delay gratification, eg doing homework before watching TV, saving money for Christmas)
o Submit to authority (parent or friendship) e.g. Adam & Eve's relationship with God is hierarchical –holding back from the tree of knowledge is a sign of that…yet they set aside that authority and choose to "become like God" themselves).

Note If we did not learn about boundaries being good for us from our parents, we might still struggle with that idea today.

Reading: Genesis 3:6 "..When the woman saw it was pleasing to the eye and also desirable she took some and ate it"

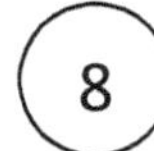 **8** **Balance in Life**
Work, living, playing and giving

Aim: To appreciate what a life balance might look like and how to develop it.

Recap: Last week's session

Icebreaker: Choose a category eg numbers 1-10 *or* types of fruit. Ask each member of the group "what am I thinking?" The object is to guess what they are not thinking and the person who guesses what the leader thought gets a fun and appropriate consequence decided by the group.

Exercise: Explain and score the WLPG sheet **over the page** and discuss.

W=Work= what we do with our working day

L=Living= what is our wider life like, our most valued relationships

P=Play= what do you do for fun, leisure, hobbies

G=Giving= what do you give unconditionally to others in terms of money or time

Making the most of my time

Life is made up of different dimensions: **Work; Living; Play; Giving**. Have a go at the WLPG questionnaire*, tick the boxes below and give yourself a score as to how you would rate each section of your life currently -5 is very high and 1 is very low.

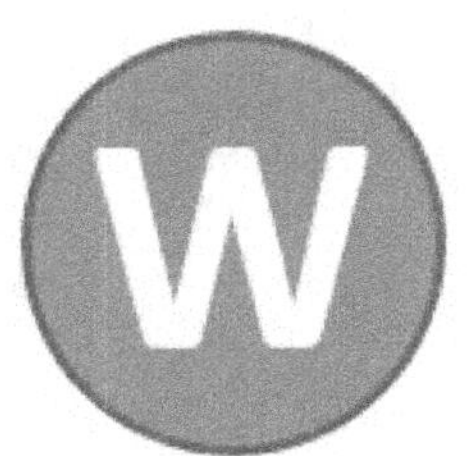

REALISING POTENTIAL How well does your work allow you to utilise your talents, gifts? How well does your work enable you to live out your faith or deepest values?

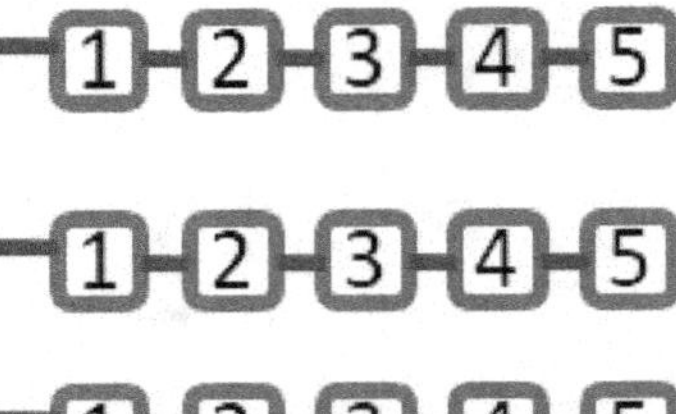

FULFILLING AND FUN Do you enjoy your work and are you passionate about it?

RECOGNITION AND REWARD Do you feel you are well rewarded for your work? (extrinsically & intrinsically)

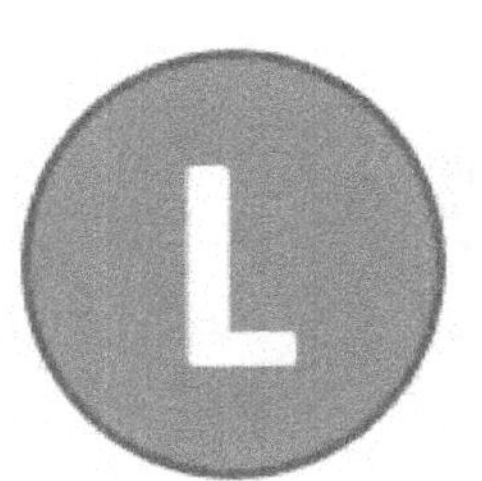

PERSONAL GROWTH How good do you feel about yourself, and your development as a person (and as a person of faith)?

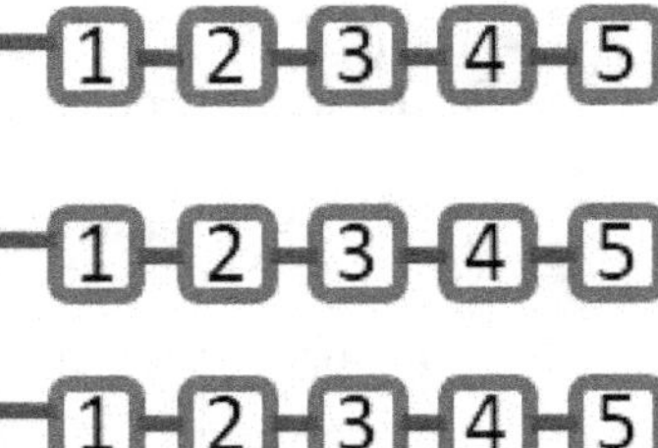

SENSE OF PURPOSE How well do your values and purpose in this life relate to those of well-being of yourself and of others near and far?

EMPLOYABILITY Do you have the right mix of skills and experience to meet any future work challenge?

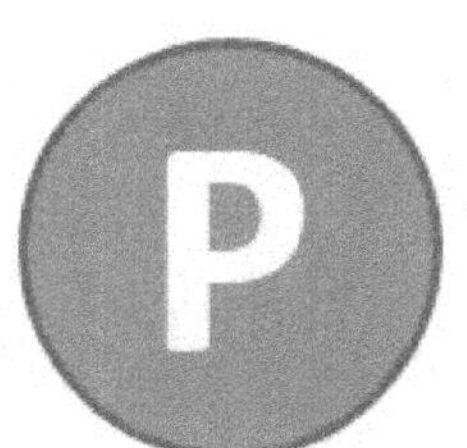

PERSONAL WELL-BEING Are you allowing yourself enough time to rest/relax? How much quality time and commitment are you giving to growing your well-being (or your relationship with God?)

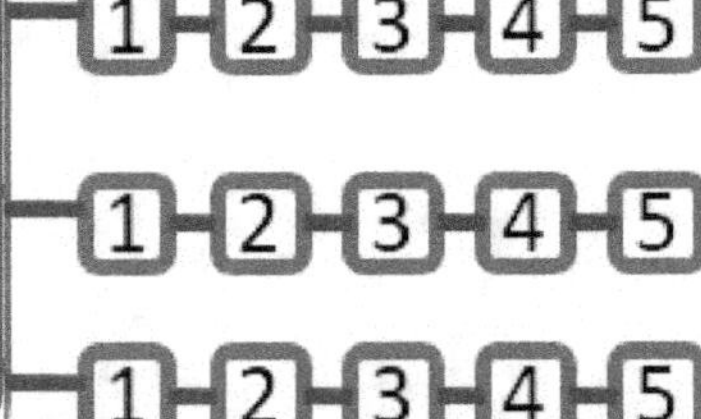

INTERESTS Do you give enough time to hobbies, sports or leisure activities that are sources of pleasure?

SOCIAL LIFE Are you giving and receiving enough help, friendship, support, love and encouragement?

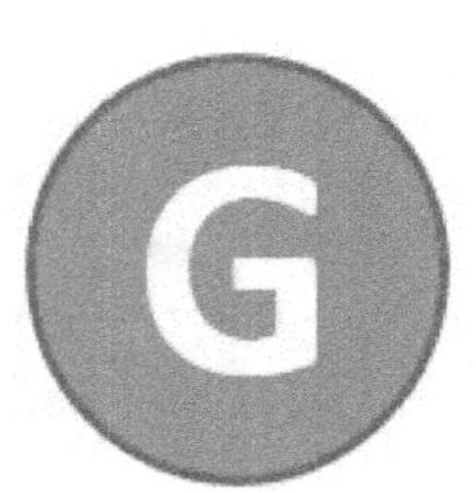

FRIENDS AND FAMILY Are you giving enough quality time, love, resources, help, friendship, support and encouragement to your close family and friends?

COMMUNITY AND ENVIRONMENT How much are you giving to improve your wider community? How much are you giving of your talents and skills for God?

UNCONDITIONAL GENEROSITY How much do you give to people and projects at home and abroad, particularly where you expect no reward or return?

When completed, consider: Where do you score highly? Are there areas for development? What are the problems and barriers that need to be addressed? Do you see possible solutions and what are your intentions?

Further work: Consider whether there is any overlap of WLPG by drawing each as a circle that intersects with the other WLPG dimensions.

*acknowledgements to www.windmillsonline.co.uk

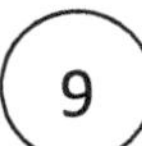

9 — Managing Money
...the love of money

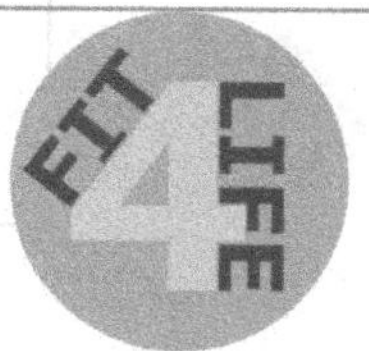

Aim: To appreciate our attitude to money can be healthy or unhealthy

Recap: Last week's session

Icebreaker: Get the group to write down on a small piece of paper answers to each of these questions. Fold each answer up and put it in the bowl. Then get each member to take an answer and guess who wrote it. Questions; Where were you brought up?/What's your favourite colour/food?/Where is the furthest place you've ever travelled?/ What is your favourite film?/ What were you doing at 8pm last night?

Discuss : "Is money good or bad?" –neither, it's neutral. It's our attitude to money that is good or bad.

Exercises:
1) Complete the Spender Saver survey* below.

-Who is in control– you or the money?

-Having a goal. What are good financial goals? -Delay gratification.

*acknowledgements to CAP (Christians Against Poverty Debt Counselling)

2) Budgets –friend or foe?
Label a number of stones with typical monthly expenses (see pic) and fill a bowl with water (pref coloured with food colouring). Get the group to place the stone one at a time into the bowl of water. Keep back the two biggest stones of Rent and Groceries. When the final two stones are revealed and put in they should stick out of the water illustrating that the water (representing our month's money) does not cover the expenses. Then start the exercise again but starting with the big stones first. This should enable more of the stones to be covered by the water illustrating if we plan, our money covers more.

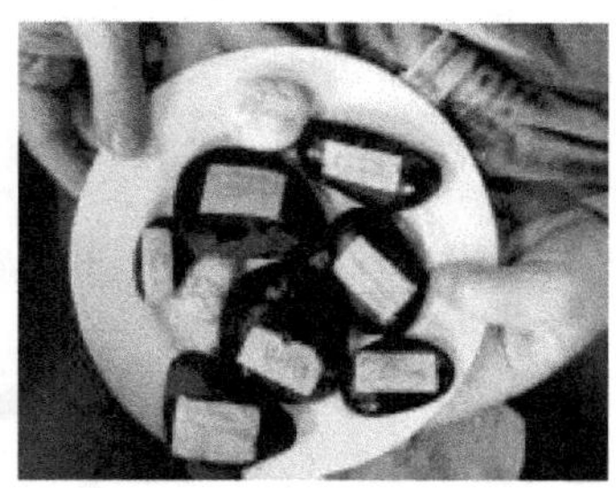

*A budget can be a pain but it sets you free -Tips for making it balance: -cut costs/cut down/cut out (cheaper = phone, utility bills; less=takeaways; or stop!) -Cash or plastic? Cash is proven to be easier to manage because it's more visible to us and easier to keep track of. -Another highly recommended tip is the "3 account system": 3 accounts for i) regular payments ii) cash account iii)savings & annual payments -If the budget doesn't balance, go for help – CAB, CAP, HOOT Credit Union **but not** pay day loans (Find your local CAP centre: www.capuk.org)*

1-20: **Spend-a-lot**: You love spending your money on things quickly and often spontaneously. Be careful to spend within your means. Spontaneity isn't a bad thing, as long as you have a fund set aside for 'spontaneous spending'

21-40: **On the spending side**: You usually succumb to 'impulse buys' but there is a part of you that sometimes stops you before you hand the money over!

41-60: **Good balance**: You are planned but your planning restrict you from making quick financial decisions. Just make sure you stick to your budget and you'll be fine

61-80: **On the saving side**: You enjoy seeing those savings build up and would rather sacrifice a short-term gain for your long-term plan. You sometimes act spontaneously, so factor this in when building your budget

81-100: **Super-saver**: You love to save every penny. It's great to be wise with your money, but don't limit your generosity or stop yourself enjoying your life whilst you save!

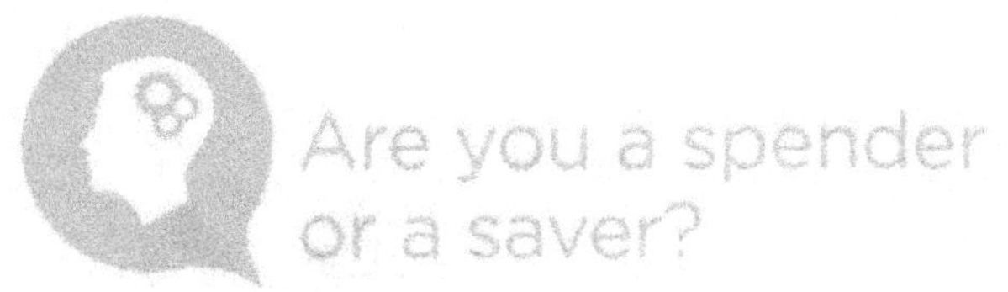

Are you a spender or a saver?

Everyone has different spending habits. Knowing whether you lean towards being more of a spender or a saver can be helpful as you prepare to look at your finances.

There are pros and cons to each spending type. Do the quiz and discuss your results.

Read each statement and tick the box that most applies to you, then add up your score.

		Always	Often	Sometimes	Rarely	Never
1	When I do my food shop I buy whatever takes my fancy	1 ☐	2 ☐	3 ☐	4 ☐	5 ☐
2	I love to buy myself a treat at the end of a hard day	1 ☐	2 ☐	3 ☐	4 ☐	5 ☐
3	I have spare cash in my purse/wallet	5 ☐	4 ☐	3 ☐	2 ☐	1 ☐
4	I borrow from my friends and family	1 ☐	2 ☐	3 ☐	4 ☐	5 ☐
5	I love to work on my budget – making tweaks where needed	5 ☐	4 ☐	3 ☐	2 ☐	1 ☐
6	Impulse buying is a weakness of mine	1 ☐	2 ☐	3 ☐	4 ☐	5 ☐
7	I prefer to stay at home in the evenings so that I don't spend any money	5 ☐	4 ☐	3 ☐	2 ☐	1 ☐
8	I find it hard to keep paying off my credit card	1 ☐	2 ☐	3 ☐	4 ☐	5 ☐
9	I make sure I have a voucher when I go out for a meal	5 ☐	4 ☐	3 ☐	2 ☐	1 ☐
10	I only spend money that I've saved, it feels very satisfying	5 ☐	4 ☐	3 ☐	2 ☐	1 ☐
11	Once I start shopping I just can't stop	1 ☐	2 ☐	3 ☐	4 ☐	5 ☐
12	I have multiple store cards	1 ☐	2 ☐	3 ☐	4 ☐	5 ☐
13	If I got a bonus at work, I would spend it straight away	1 ☐	2 ☐	3 ☐	4 ☐	5 ☐
14	I feel satisfied when I see my bank balance grow	5 ☐	4 ☐	3 ☐	2 ☐	1 ☐
15	I feel that it's worth spending my money on luxury items	1 ☐	2 ☐	3 ☐	4 ☐	5 ☐
16	I find it difficult to spend on people when Christmas comes around	5 ☐	4 ☐	3 ☐	2 ☐	1 ☐
17	I love shopping in second hand shops – you can find so many bargains	5 ☐	4 ☐	3 ☐	2 ☐	1 ☐
18	I only buy something when I know I need it	5 ☐	4 ☐	3 ☐	2 ☐	1 ☐
19	Money is there for me to bring happiness to myself and others	1 ☐	2 ☐	3 ☐	4 ☐	5 ☐
20	I make sure that I have savings for my long-term future	5 ☐	4 ☐	3 ☐	2 ☐	1 ☐

Total score: ☐

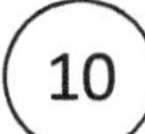

(10)   **Goals**
...the power of setting them

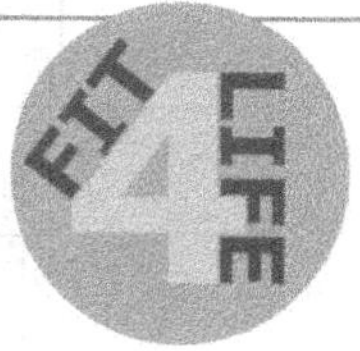

Aim: To appreciate how setting goals can help you make progress

Recap: Last week's session

Icebreaker: Ask people to score how they feel out of ten (remembering Banksy's picture). Then ask them to give one word (if possible) to explain why they scored their feelings with that number. This is a recommended icebreaker for every session.

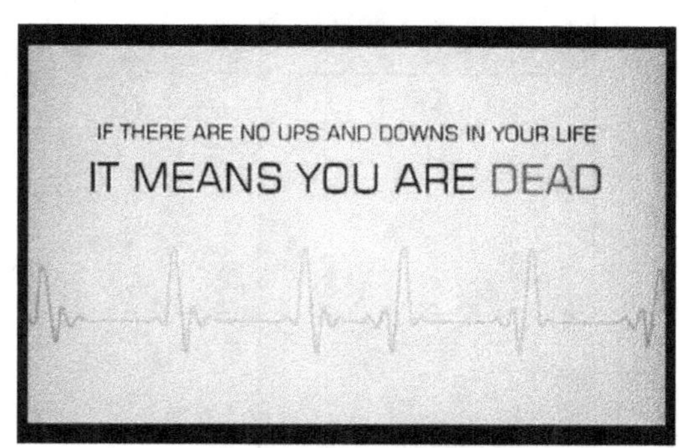

Discuss : one or both of these quotes *"Give me a stock clerk with a goal and I'll give you a man who will make history. Give me a man with no goals and I'll give you a stock clerk." JC Penny (Founder of Penny Stores USA) "By looking at your diary this week it is possible to predict where you will be in 3-5 years time" (-the idea that our big goals are made up of lots of small goals that we have to be committed to)*

Exercise: Discuss the Rule of Life Grid below. Spend some time completing the Rule of Life Grid and share if you can. Try to put an action or activity, in each box, that you can do at these different frequencies with these different contexts.

Personal Rule of Life Grid. Name:________________

	Personal	Family	Friends	Club/ Church/ Community	Working Day	Leisure time	Relaxation/ Retreat
Daily							
Weekly							
Monthly							
Annually							

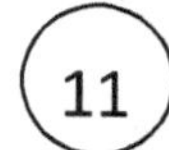

(11) Healthy Relationships –Part 1
....why is staying together so hard?

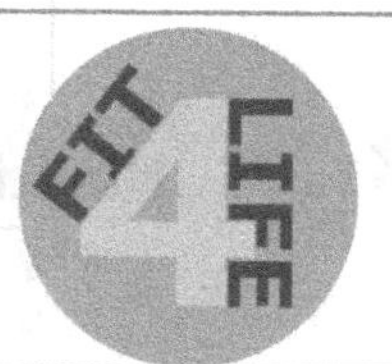

Aim: To appreciate how some of the obstacles to healthy relationships in the family might be overcome.

Relationships Factfile:
40% of couples living together break up by the time their first child is 5. Children with an absent father (figs below from Carl Beech CVM.org)
o Suicide x5 higher
o Runaway from home x32 higher
o Rape x14 higher
o Drop out of ed x9 higher
o Drugs x10 higher
o Prison x20 higher

Discussion: Why is staying together so hard?....
3 major areas of difference that we need to deal with rather than fight or run away from;
1) *Histories & Futures*

Question: What do you think the top 5 things women look for in men and vice-versa.
His needs:
• Sexual fulfilment
• Recreational companionship
• An attractive spouse
• Domestic support
• Admiration from his wife
Her needs:
• Affection
• Conversation
• Honesty & openness
• Financial support
• Family commitment

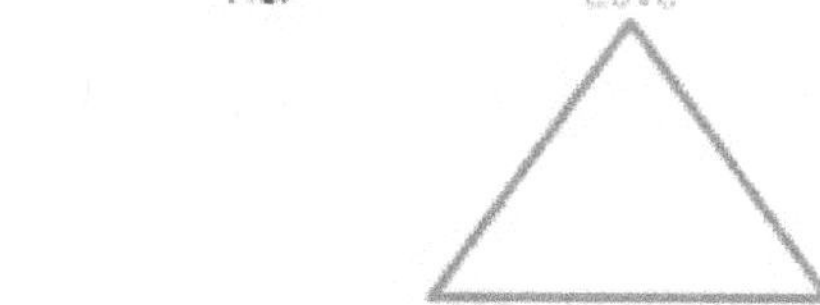

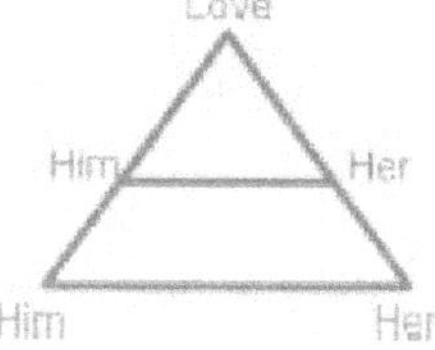

2) Personalities:
Myers-Briggs indicator shows types such as introvert–extrovert, intuitive-analytical, etc. These are personality traits that come from the "inner onion layers" and may affect the outer layers of us e.g. the way we dress.
Question: What is your personality - introvert–extrovert?

3) Communication
Active Listening skills Discussion: "God gave us 2 ears and 1 mouth for a reason".
-Experts say there are 5 "Love Languages": Physical affection; Kind Actions; Thoughtful Presents; Quality Time; Loving Words
Question: What is your "love language"?
-Saying sorry & I forgive is important communication

Discussion: Is compromise the key to dealing with differences? See Diagram above: *Compromise can create a dynamic of "giving in" to control of the other- like a tug of war. Whereas focussing on sacrificial love causes us to put the other first and creates a dynamic of bringing us together. As we grow in sacrificial love, we grow closer together.*

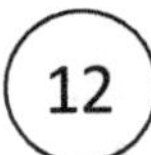

(12) Healthy Relationships –Part 2
....why is work such a nightmare?

Aim: To appreciate how some of the obstacles to healthy relationships in the workplace might be overcome.

Relationships Factfile:
50% of people leave their job because they don't like their boss.
Well-managed workgroups are more profitable (44% higher), more productive (50% higher), and have higher degrees of customer loyalty (50% higher).

Discuss: what does "well managed" look like?
Gallup has studied more than one million employees across hundreds of organizations and has identified the 12 elements of good management (see next page);
Which of the 12 is most important to you – why? -How can we influence these things happening in our workplace?
-Is there anything else that is important in the workplace?

Discuss: -Which 3 of these "7 Laws" for success would you prioritise?
(Rob Parsons – The Heart of Success)
1) Don't settle for being "money rich-time poor"
2) Believe that the job you do makes a difference
3) Play to your strengths-Find your X factor
4) Believe in the power of dreams
5) Put your family before your career
6) Keep the common touch
7) Don't settle for success: Make a difference, Strive for significance

Personality:

Using this model, try and identify which personality ABCD describes you best?

Each personality offers a unique strength to teams. What are they?

Which personality do you find the hardest to work with and why?

Parents often find their children are different personalities to themselves. How might we modify our behaviour for the sake of encouraging other personalities.

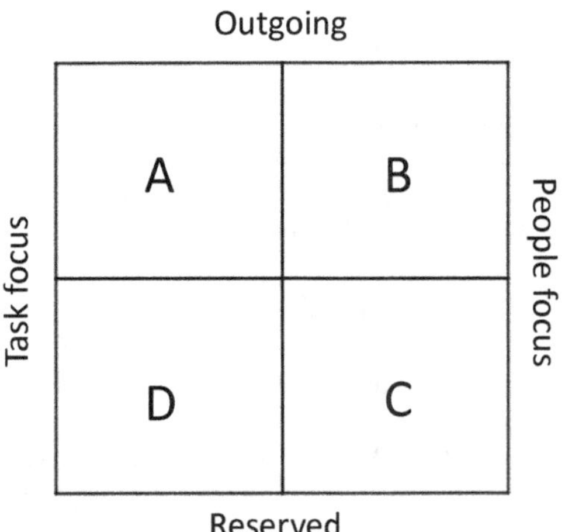

The 12 Elements of Great Managing

To identify the elements of worker engagement, Gallup conducted many thousands of interviews in all kinds of organizations, at all levels, in most industries, and in many countries. These 12 statements – the Gallup Q^{12} – emerged from Gallup's pioneering research as those that best predict employee and workgroup performance.

1. I know what is expected of me at work.

2. I have the materials and equipment I need to do my work right.

3. At work, I have the opportunity to do what I do best every day.

4. In the last seven days, I have received recognition or praise for doing good work.

5. My supervisor, or someone at work, seems to care about me as a person.

6. There is someone at work who encourages my development.

7. At work, my opinions seem to count.

8. The mission or purpose of my company makes me feel my job is important.

9. My associates or fellow employees are committed to doing quality work.

10. I have a best friend at work.

11. In the last six months, someone at work has talked to me about my progress.

12. This last year, I have had opportunities at work to learn and grow.

Read: 1 Corinthians 13 in the Bible

ABOUT THE AUTHOR

Mark Cowling has worked as a Church of England minister since 2007 and is the founder of Third Space Bolton, a charity that supports wellbeing of young people. Prior to 2007, Mark worked in the medical industry based in the UK, Australia and Ireland. He is married to Rachel and they have three children.

Any profits from the sales of this book will be given to the work of supporting, inspiring and uniting young people.